UNDERSTANDING

COENZYME Q10

AND BENEFITS

A Comprehensive Guide to Targeting Cellular Energy, for Heart Health, Energy, and Anti-Aging

DR. LACEY MICHELLE

Disclaimer:

The information provided in this book is for general informational purposes only and is not intended as medical advice.

Readers are encouraged to consult with a qualified healthcare professional for any health concerns or questions.

The author of this book is not affiliated with any individual, website, organization, or products mentioned within.

This book does not endorse or promote any specific brands, services, or external entities. Any references made are purely for illustrative purposes and should not be construed as endorsements.

Readers are responsible for their own decisions and should conduct their own research before making any health-related choices.

Any liability resulting from the use of this information, whether direct or indirect, is disclaimed by the author and publisher.

Contents

About The Book

Comprehending Coenzyme Q10

Coenzyme Q10, often known as CoQ10, is an essential substance that is crucial to preserving general health. This section delves into the fundamentals of Coenzyme Q10, examining its composition, roles, and importance inside the body. We also look at the different ways that our bodies get this vital coenzyme.

Fundamentals of Coenzyme Q10

A naturally occurring coenzyme, coenzyme Q10 is essential to the body's process of generating energy. We learn about the chemical details of CoQ10 and its role in the synthesis of adenosine triphosphate (ATP), our cells' main source of energy. Comprehending its composition and operation serves as the basis for appreciating its wider health consequences.

The Body's Coenzyme Q10

In this section, we look at the distribution of Coenzyme Q10 in the human body, as well as the organs and tissues that depend on it for vital functions. Further investigation of CoQ10's health effects is made possible by its association with cellular energy production and its presence in multiple body systems.

Where to Find Coenzyme Q10

We look into how Coenzyme Q10 comes from both internal and external sources. This section explains the processes by which we obtain this coenzyme and sustain optimal levels of CoQ10, ranging from dietary intake to endogenous production.

Health Advantages

The Heart and Coenzyme Q10

As we learn more about the critical function Coenzyme Q10 plays in cardiovascular health, heart health becomes increasingly important. We explore the possible advantages of CoQ10 in preserving cardiac health and talk about its consequences for people who are at risk of developing heart-related disorders.

Coenzyme Q10 as a Protective Agent

This section examines the antioxidant qualities of CoQ10, highlighting its ability to fend off oxidative stress and shield cells from harm. We explore how the antioxidant properties of Coenzyme Q10 support general health and well-being.

Coenzyme Q10 for vigor and endurance

Vitality and endurance are essential elements of our everyday existence. The impact of CoQ10 on energy metabolism and its capacity to increase endurance are discussed. This section offers information on how Coenzyme Q10 could improve athletic performance.

Skin Health and Coenzyme Q10

In addition to being an internal powerhouse, coenzyme Q10 may also improve our outward look. We explore the possible benefits of CoQ10 as a skincare supplement and how it can improve skin health.

Coenzyme Q10 for Mental Wellness

Maintaining cognitive health is crucial. We investigate the connections between Coenzyme Q10 and brain health, highlighting its contribution to maintaining cognitive health and possibly preventing age-related cognitive decline.

Q10 Coenzyme and Immune Boosting

In this section, we explore the possible effects of CoQ10 on the immune system with a particular emphasis on immunological support. We look at the potential benefits of Coenzyme Q10 for enhancing the body's defenses and promoting general health.

Vitamin Q10 in Exercise and Sports

The role that Coenzyme Q10 plays in maximizing physical performance for people who participate in sports and fitness is examined. We explore its possible advantages for athletes and physically active people.

Adding Coenzyme Q10 as a Supplement

The Best Coenzyme Q10 Supplement to Take

Choosing the best Coenzyme Q10 supplement is essential, and this section provides advice on how to do so. We go over the various kinds of CoQ10 and things to think about when choosing a supplement.

Guidelines for Dosage and Usage

This section covers suggestions for optimal dosage and usage. We offer suggestions on how to optimize the health advantages of CoQ10 by incorporating it into your daily routine.

Possible Adverse Reactions and Concurrent Events

We discuss possible side effects and interactions that people should be aware of while using Coenzyme Q10 as a dietary supplement because safety is the priority when it comes to Coenzyme Q10 consumption.

Coenzyme Q10 for Particular Illnesses

This section looks at how Coenzyme Q10 may be used to treat various medical disorders, including diabetes, heart disease, and more. We go over the studies that back up CoQ10's ability to control and enhance various ailments.

Way of Life and Coenzyme Q10

Diet and Q10 Coenzyme

Coenzyme Q10 levels can be significantly impacted by dietary decisions. We go over how your diet can affect the amount of CoQ10 you consume as well as how to include foods high in Coenzyme Q10 in your meals.

Lifestyle Elements to Optimize the Benefits of Coenzyme Q10

Choosing the right lifestyle is also essential to maximizing the health advantages of CoQ10. We investigate the relationship between Coenzyme Q10 levels and general health and variables such as stress, exercise, and sleep.

Research and Upcoming Projects

Current Coenzyme Q10 Research

This section presents the most recent Coenzyme Q10 research findings as well as current projects. We go over the state of science's knowledge on CoQ10's health advantages as well as possible future advancements.

Prospects for Future Growth and Opportunities

We consider the promising prospects and future paths in the study of Coenzyme Q10 and its contribution to improving health and well-being. We examine future discoveries and breakthroughs that might occur.

In summary

The complex role that Coenzyme Q10 plays in enhancing general health is summed up in the final section. It highlights how utilizing CoQ10 to its full potential can be a beneficial part of your journey toward better health. For those seeking heart health, cognitive assistance, increased energy, or other benefits, Coenzyme Q10 is a flexible and promising vitamin that can help them achieve optimal health.

CHAPTER ONE

Knowledge Of Coenzyme Q10

Fundamentals Of Coenzyme Q10

Coenzyme Q10, or CoQ10, is a necessary substance that is present in the human body. It is also a strong antioxidant and plays a critical part in the synthesis of cellular energy.

Though it has a structure similar to a vitamin, CoQ10 is a fat-soluble molecule that is categorized as a coenzyme. The body can generate modest amounts of it, and it can also be acquired through diet and supplementation.

The mitochondria, our cells' energy-producing powerhouses, are where CoQ10 is mostly found. There are two forms of the compound: ubiquinone and ubiquinol. The more popular supplemental form is ubiquinone.

Coenzyme Q10's Function In The Body

Participating in the electron transport chain, a vital step in cellular respiration that yields adenosine triphosphate (ATP), the molecule that stores and transports energy within cells, is the main job of coenzyme Q10.

The body produces less ATP when CoQ10 levels are insufficient, which lowers energy levels. This is especially crucial for organs like the heart, liver, and muscles that have significant energy requirements. CoQ10 is very important for the heart since it keeps pounding constantly.

Moreover, CoQ10 acts as a potent antioxidant, preventing oxidative damage to lipids and cells. Free radicals are unstable chemicals linked to aging, sickness, and cellular damage that are neutralized by this substance. CoQ10 fights oxidative stress in the body by collaborating with other antioxidants, such as vitamins C and E.

Additionally, studies have indicated that Coenzyme Q10 may be beneficial in the treatment of several illnesses.

 For example, its potential to boost cardiovascular health by lowering blood pressure and improving cholesterol profiles has been investigated. Furthermore, CoQ10 has been studied in the treatment of illnesses related to the mitochondria, where a shortage can cause weariness and weakening in the muscles. Research on its potential to treat ailments like diabetes, Parkinson's disease, and migraines is still ongoing; however, more data is required to prove any firm therapeutic advantages.

Coenzyme Q10 Supplement Types

Various types of Coenzyme Q10 can be purchased as dietary supplements. There are two main types: ubiquinone and ubiquinol. The oxidized form of CoQ10 is called ubiquinone, while the reduced form is called ubiquinol.

The more common and stable form found in most foods and supplements is ubiquinone. The body changes ubiquinone into ubiquinol upon ingestion so that it can be utilized in cellular functions.

However, some people may benefit from taking ubiquinol supplements straight, particularly those with disorders that impair their capacity to convert ubiquinone to ubiquinol.

CoQ10 supplements come in a variety of forms, such as liquids, soft gels, and capsules, and are generally accessible over the counter.

Depending on the intended use, different dosages may be advised; for general health maintenance, common doses range from 100 to 300 milligrams per day.

Higher dosages, however, might be necessary for people seeking therapeutic advantages or for those with particular health issues; this should be discussed with a healthcare provider.

For the synthesis of cellular energy and as an antioxidant, coenzyme Q10 is an essential substance.

It has a variety of functions in the body, including protecting cells from oxidative stress and supplying energy to the mitochondria. CoQ10 supplements, which come in ubiquinone and ubiquinol forms, have been the focus of scientific research on several medical disorders and may have health advantages.

When thinking about taking CoQ10 supplements, it's best to speak with a doctor to figure out the best dosage and form depending on your unique needs and health objectives.

CHAPTER TWO

Advantages Of Coenzyme Q10 For Health

Heart Health: Coenzyme Q10 (CoQ10), sometimes referred to as ubiquinone, is essential for preserving cardiovascular health. It plays a crucial role in the electron transport chain, which makes adenosine triphosphate (ATP), the body's main energy source, easier to produce. CoQ10 promotes heart health by boosting the cardiac muscle's ability to produce energy.

As a supplement, it has been thoroughly investigated for people with cardiac diseases, including hypertension, angina, and heart failure. CoQ10 is a useful supplement to cardiac treatment since it is thought to raise heart rate, lower blood pressure, and improve cardiac function.

The body uses CoQ10 as a necessary component to produce energy. It assists in converting dietary energy into ATP by taking part in the mitochondrial electron transport cycle.

This function is especially important for muscles that need a lot of energy to work properly, like the heart. Consequently, those wishing to improve their general energy and stamina may find that taking a CoQ10 supplement helps. CoQ10 has been investigated by athletes and those suffering from chronic fatigue syndrome as a way to increase their energy stores.

Antioxidant Properties: The body uses CoQ10 as a strong antioxidant as well. As an antioxidant, it aids in preventing the damaging effects of free radicals, which are unstable molecules that can lead to oxidative stress and cellular damage. CoQ10 may lower the risk of chronic diseases like cancer, heart disease, and neurological disorders by scavenging free radicals. Antioxidant activity has the potential to improve general health and wellness.

Cognitive Function: Studies on CoQ10 have looked into how it might affect mental health and cognitive function. Given how dependent the brain is on energy, CoQ10's function in energy synthesis may have an impact on cognitive function.

Supplementing with CoQ10 may aid those suffering from cognitive decline, neurodegenerative disorders like Alzheimer's, or other ailments that impact brain function with their memory, cognition, and mood, according to certain studies.

Skin Health: The advantages of CoQ10 for skin health are becoming more well-acknowledged.

Wrinkles and other aging symptoms are caused by oxidative stress and decreased collagen formation in the skin as we age. Because CoQ10 is an antioxidant, it may be able to slow down the aging process by shielding the skin from UV radiation and free radical damage.

It is a beneficial supplement to skincare regimens because it may also help with skin regeneration and healing.

Possible Weight control: CoQ10 might help with weight control, even if it's not a magic pill for weight loss. It may assist in increasing metabolism and decreasing body fat, according to some research; however, more research is required to establish these benefits. Its ability to increase energy may indirectly help with weight management by encouraging physical activity and lowering weariness.

Additional Potential Benefits: CoQ10 has demonstrated potential in several other areas of health. For example, enhancing blood sugar regulation might help with diabetic management.

According to some research, CoQ10 may help people with migraines by lessening the frequency and intensity of their attacks. Furthermore, the possible effect of CoQ10 in promoting male reproductive health and fertility is being investigated. Furthermore, it might mitigate the negative effects of some drugs, including statins, which lower the body's levels of CoQ10.

Coenzyme Q10 is an amazing substance that has several possible health advantages. CoQ10 has gained a lot of attention in the dietary supplement industry for its many benefits, including heart health, energy production, and skin, cognitive, and weight management benefits as well as its role as an antioxidant.

Before adding CoQ10 to your daily regimen, you should, however, speak with a healthcare provider because each person's demands and responses are unique and the right amount and usage may vary depending on particular health conditions or objectives.

Suggested Doses: Coenzyme Q10, or CoQ10, is an essential coenzyme that the body naturally produces and is essential to the cellular synthesis of energy. Additionally, it functions as a strong antioxidant, shielding cells from harm brought on by dangerous free radicals. Because of its possible health advantages, CoQ10 has become more and more popular as a dietary supplement. The suggested dosage of CoQ10 can change based on a person's needs and medical history.

 For most healthy adults, a daily dosage of 100–200 mg is generally regarded as typical. Nevertheless, dosages can vary from thirty milligrams to 600 milligrams or more, contingent upon the need for supplementation and an individual's particular health objectives.

Coenzyme Q10 in Various Types: Ubiquinone and ubiquinol are two of the types of CoQ10 supplements that are available. The reduced, active form of CoQ10 is called ubiquinol, whereas its oxidized version is called ubiquinone.

Both ubiquinone and ubiquinol have advantages since the body can convert them into one another. While ubiquinol is frequently thought to be the more accessible form, ubiquinone is more frequently encountered in supplements and is thought to be stable.

Selecting The Form That Best Fits Your Requirements And Tastes Is Crucial.

Furthermore, CoQ10 is available in a variety of dosage forms, including chewable tablets, soft gels, and capsules. Several considerations, including convenience, dietary constraints, and absorption rates, may influence the choice of form and delivery mechanism.

When and How to Take Coenzyme Q10: The best time to take a CoQ10 supplement will depend on its efficacy. Since CoQ10 is a fat-soluble substance, it is best absorbed when consumed with meals that have some fat in the diet. The bioavailability of CoQ10 can be increased by taking it with a meal that contains healthy fats, such as those in avocados or olive oil. It might also be possible to maintain more consistent levels in the bloodstream by splitting the daily intake into two or three smaller doses spaced out throughout the day.

Before beginning CoQ10 supplementation, it is imperative to speak with a healthcare provider because the right time and amount can vary according to a person's health and prescription schedule. Certain medical disorders, like heart disease, may require greater dosages or certain timing to achieve the best possible outcomes.

Combining Coenzyme Q10 with Other Supplements: As long as there are no interactions or contraindications that would jeopardize the safety or efficacy of the supplement, Coenzyme Q10 can be taken with other dietary supplements.

 Certain supplements, such as vitamin E or selenium, which both have antioxidant qualities that enhance CoQ10's ability to neutralize free radicals, may function in concert with CoQ10.

However, while using CoQ10 together with other drugs, it's important to be mindful of possible interactions. CoQ10, for instance, may interfere with drugs that thin the blood, such as warfarin, or those that treat high blood pressure. To prevent any negative effects, it is crucial to speak with a healthcare professional before using CoQ10 in addition to prescription drugs.

Coenzyme Q10 is an adaptable vitamin that may help with a variety of ailments, from energy generation to cardiovascular health. To maximize the benefits of supplements, it is crucial to comprehend the suggested dosages, types, and timing.

To ensure safety and effectiveness, it's also advisable to speak with a healthcare provider before using CoQ10 with any supplements or drugs.

Sources Of Coenzyme Q10 In Nature:

Coenzyme Q10 sometimes referred to as ubiquinone or CoQ10, is a naturally occurring substance that can be found in some foods and the human body.

This essential coenzyme functions as a strong antioxidant to shield cells from oxidative damage and is essential for the synthesis of cellular energy. CoQ10 can be produced by the body, but it can also be acquired through diet and supplementation. It's important to know where Coenzyme Q10 comes from and how it benefits general health when looking for natural sources of the vitamin.

Vitamin Q10 In Food:

There are different quantities of CoQ10 in different kinds of food. Meat, poultry, and fish are some of the main food sources of coenzyme Q10. Organ meats with the highest CoQ10 contents include the liver, heart, and kidney. Additionally, fatty fish like sardines, mackerel, and salmon are good sources of this coenzyme. It's crucial to remember that cooking and processing animal-based meals may cause their CoQ10 content to drop, therefore it's advantageous to use preparation techniques that maintain these levels. Smaller concentrations of CoQ10 are also present in certain oils, nuts, and seeds.

The fact that plants can also produce coenzyme Q10 is a fascinating feature of this substance. Cauliflower, broccoli, and spinach are a few veggies that include CoQ10. A small amount of this coenzyme can also be found in grains, such as wheat and whole grains. Even while plant-based meals often contain less CoQ10 than animal-based foods, they are still a beneficial choice for people who follow vegetarian or vegan diets.

CHAPTER THREE

Dietary Influence On Coenzyme Q10 Intake:

A major factor in determining Coenzyme Q10 intake is diet. Foods are the primary source of CoQ10 for humans, and an unbalanced or insufficient diet can result in a lack of this vital coenzyme.

Since the body can produce CoQ10, it is not regarded as an essential nutrient; however, dietary sources can increase the nutrient's total availability.

A person's requirements for CoQ10 might change based on several variables, including age, health, and physical activity.

Because of its function in the cellular generation of energy, CoQ10 may be particularly necessary for athletes and those with high energy demands.

Additionally, as the body's natural production of CoQ10 tends to decline with age, elderly people may benefit from dietary sources of the nutrient.

CoQ10 supplements are available for people who don't get enough CoQ10 from their diet or who have certain health issues.

These supplements are frequently used as antioxidants, to enhance energy levels, and to improve heart health. Before beginning any supplementation, it's crucial to speak with a healthcare provider to ascertain the right dosage and weigh the advantages and disadvantages.

Coenzyme Q10 is an essential coenzyme that is obtained from natural food sources, mostly animal foods (meat, poultry, and fish) and certain plant foods (vegetables and grains). A balanced, nutrient-rich diet can help guarantee enough amounts of this coenzyme for general health and well-being.

Diet has a crucial influence on CoQ10 intake. Under the supervision of a healthcare professional, supplements are a viable choice for individuals with particular dietary restrictions or medical issues.

Safety And Adverse Reactions

Fat-soluble Coenzyme Q10 (CoQ10) is present in almost all human cells and is essential for the synthesis of energy as well as serving as an antioxidant.

Because of its possible health benefits, CoQ10 has become more popular as a dietary supplement. However, like with any supplement, it's vital to think about safety and any negative effects.

Typical Adverse Effects

When used as prescribed, CoQ10 is usually regarded as safe. The majority of adverse effects are moderate, and they can include gastrointestinal issues like nausea, diarrhea, and upset stomach.

 By taking the supplement with food, you can frequently reduce these dose-dependent side effects. Although they are uncommon, allergic reactions to CoQ10 can happen and cause symptoms like swelling, redness, and itching.

It is advised to stop using the medication and see a doctor if you have severe or ongoing negative effects.

CoQ10 is typically safe, but there are some guidelines and caveats to be aware of. Because there is little information on the safety of CoQ10 supplements during pregnancy and lactation, women who are pregnant or nursing should speak with their healthcare professional before using these supplements.

Before beginning CoQ10 supplementation, anyone with pre-existing medical issues, particularly those with heart disease, diabetes, or low blood pressure, should speak with their healthcare professional because CoQ10 may interfere with medication and treatment regimens.

CoQ10 supplements should be used with caution by anyone using blood-thinning medications, such as warfarin (Coumadin), or antiplatelet medications, as they may interfere and raise the risk of bleeding.

Additionally, CoQ10 can lower blood sugar levels, so if a diabetic taking medicine to regulate their blood sugar chooses to take CoQ10, they should regularly monitor their blood glucose levels.

Interactions Between Drugs

CoQ10 and other drugs may interact, which could reduce their efficacy or have unfavorable effects. CoQ10 may interact with pharmaceuticals such as beta-blockers, certain chemotherapeutic agents, antipsychotic meds, and the previously mentioned blood-thinning and diabetic therapies.

It's critical to let your doctor know about all of the supplements you take to prevent any potential interactions and to modify your treatment plan as needed.

Particular Populations

Supplementing with CoQ10 may have particular advantages for certain groups of people, such as athletes, older adults, and people with particular medical issues.

Due to a natural decrease in CoQ10 levels with age, older persons may benefit from CoQ10, which may aid in energy generation and general vigor.

CoQ10 may help athletes and physically active people increase their endurance and speed up their recovery times, but there isn't much data to support these claims.

Under the supervision of a healthcare provider, those with particular medical issues, such as heart disease, migraines, and some genetic abnormalities, may also think about taking CoQ10 supplements. CoQ10 may be able to help control symptoms and enhance quality of life in several situations.

Supplementing with coenzyme Q10 may have health benefits, but users should be aware of possible drug combinations, typical side effects, precautions, safety issues, and their unique requirements based on age, health, and activity level.

 Before beginning any new supplement regimen, including CoQ10, it is always advisable to speak with a healthcare professional to make sure it is safe and suitable for your particular situation.

CHAPTER FOUR

Selecting A Supplemental Coenzyme Q10:

Making an informed decision is crucial when thinking about using a Coenzyme Q10 (CoQ10) supplement to make sure you're obtaining a high-quality product that suits your individual needs.

The body naturally produces CoQ10, which is an essential component of cell energy generation. It also has strong antioxidant properties that shield cells from oxidative harm. Although our bodies are capable of producing CoQ10, age, and certain medical problems might cause our bodies to produce less of this essential substance, so taking supplements may be a good alternative.

What Makes A Quality Supplement What It Is:

Choosing a premium CoQ10 supplement is essential to guaranteeing both its efficacy and safety. The following are important things to think about while selecting a CoQ10 supplement:

CoQ10 Form: Ubiquinone and ubiquinol are the two main forms of CoQ10 that supplements are available in. The more prevalent form is ubiquinone, which the body can change into ubiquinol as necessary. Since ubiquinol is already in its active form, it might be a better option for people, such as elderly people, who have trouble converting ubiquinone. Which of these two types is best for you may depend on your health demands.

Purity and Potency: Verify the CoQ10 supplement's potency and purity. A superior product has to be devoid of impurities and offer the specified quantity of CoQ10 for each serving. Seek supplements that have their purity and quality evaluated by a third party.

Bioavailability: Because CoQ10 is a fat-soluble substance, it is best absorbed when consumed with a meal that includes some good fats. Certain CoQ10 supplements have been designed to increase their bioavailability, which means that the body will be able to absorb them more efficiently.

amount: Depending on a person's unique health objectives and requirements, there are differences in the recommended amount of CoQ10. The appropriate dosage for your circumstances should be determined by speaking with a healthcare provider. A larger intake may be necessary in certain situations, while a smaller amount might be adequate in others.

Value and Cost: Take into account the supplement's total worth as well as the cost per serving. Not all products that cost more are better, so be sure to weigh the price against the quantity and quality of CoQ10 that is offered.

Additives and Fillers: Carefully review the ingredient list to make sure the supplement doesn't include any unneeded additives, fillers, or allergies. Choose items that don't contain a lot of extra components.

Various Shapes And Labels:

CoQ10 supplements are available from many different companies and in different formats. As previously stated, the decision between ubiquinone and ubiquinol is based on your unique requirements. Fast-absorbing and extended-release versions are also available. CoQ10 may also be included by certain manufacturers in combination supplements that also contain antioxidants, other vitamins, and minerals.

Choosing the appropriate form and brand is an individual choice. It's critical to take into account elements like your food choices, practicality, and any particular health issues you may be experiencing. Examine various brands and read reviews to determine how well-regarded they are for efficacy and quality.

Examining Certifications And Labels:
It is essential to study the labels for CoQ10 supplements to make an informed decision. Seek for the following details:

Serving Size: The suggested serving size and the quantity of servings per container should be made crystal clear on the label.

CoQ10 Content: The amount of CoQ10 per serving, usually expressed in milligrams (mg), should be listed on the label. If a healthcare provider has advised it, make sure the dosage is the same as what you are prescribed.

Ingredients: Go over the ingredient list carefully to be sure there are no fillers, unneeded additions, or possible allergens that you want to stay away from.

Storage Recommendations: To preserve their effectiveness, certain CoQ10 supplements may need to be kept in a particular environment, such as cold storage.

Certifications: Seek certifications attesting to the product's quality and purity from respectable third-party organizations, such as ConsumerLab.com or the United States Pharmacopeia (USP).

When selecting a Coenzyme Q10 supplement, you should carefully consider your unique requirements and preferences in addition to carefully examining the product's quality, purity, and label information. When in doubt, it's a good idea to speak with a medical expert for tailored advice on which CoQ10 supplement is best for your particular health objectives.

Studies And Verifiable Science:

Every human cell contains the naturally occurring substance coenzyme Q10 (CoQ10), commonly referred to as ubiquinone. It is a strong antioxidant and is essential for the synthesis of adenosine triphosphate (ATP), which is the energy source. CoQ10 is mostly produced in the mitochondria and is essential for many different biological functions, especially those that demand a lot of energy. CoQ10 has drawn a lot of attention as a dietary supplement due to its possible health advantages. Over the years, a wealth of scientific data and significant research have been gathered to help understand the effectiveness and effects of CoQ10 supplementation.

Clinical Research And Experiments:

Several clinical trials and research have investigated the impact of CoQ10 supplementation on a range of medical disorders. The treatment of heart-related conditions is one of the most well-established uses of CoQ10. For example, studies have demonstrated that CoQ10 can lower blood pressure and help individuals with heart failure feel better.

 In addition, CoQ10 has been studied in cardiovascular illness, where it may help lower the likelihood of unfavorable outcomes, such as heart attacks.

The potential advantages of CoQ10 go beyond cardiovascular health. Research has looked into its application in neurological disorders like Alzheimer's and Parkinson's disease.

Although further investigation is required to determine its exact function, CoQ10 has demonstrated the potential to shield brain cells from oxidative stress and injury.

Furthermore, CoQ10 has been researched for its ability to enhance fertility and treat male infertility problems.

CoQ10 supplementation may improve sperm motility and quality, which may improve reproductive results, according to research.

CoQ10's antioxidant qualities have been recognized in the fields of dermatology and skincare for their ability to minimize the effects of aging and shield the skin from UV damage. It's a useful element in topical applications because of its capacity to counteract free radicals.

Notwithstanding these encouraging results, it's crucial to remember that CoQ10 study outcomes can differ and that advantages from clinical trials haven't always been consistently reported.

Results can be affected by variables like dosage, formulation, and the particular medical problem under investigation. Consequently, further study is necessary to comprehend the best application of CoQ10 in diverse settings.

The Prospects For Research On Coenzyme Q10:

Coenzyme Q10 research has promising potential for the future. Researchers are expected to find new applications and improve ones that already exist as our understanding of its molecular principles and potential advantages grows. Personalized medicine presents a promising path for investigating how CoQ10 usage might be customized to an individual's own genetic and health profile.

The development of formulation methods and drug delivery systems may potentially be crucial to the direction of CoQ10 research. Better ways to distribute CoQ10, including liposomal or nanoparticle formulations, may increase its bioavailability and effectiveness, increasing its potency in a range of therapeutic and medicinal uses.

Additionally, scientists will keep looking at how CoQ10 interacts with other substances, including how it works in concert with other nutrients and antioxidants.

This cooperative strategy could result in the creation of innovative combination treatments with improved health advantages.

Coenzyme Q10 research is positioned to play a crucial role in the ongoing evolution of the health and wellness industry.

Because of its ability to affect many facets of human health, such as anti-aging tactics and cardiovascular health, scientists are always working to fully understand its therapeutic potential.

As more research is conducted and clinical trials continue, CoQ10 is expected to continue to be recognized as an effective and adaptable supplement that supports health and vigor.

CHAPTER FIVE

Including Coenzyme Q10 In Your Daily Diet

Coenzyme Q10, or CoQ10 as it is more well known, is a substance that exists naturally in human cells. It is essential for the synthesis of energy and serves as an antioxidant. CoQ10 is essential for preserving general health, and certain medical disorders or aging might cause a decrease in its levels. Many possible benefits can be obtained by including CoQ10 in your diet, but it's important to do so sensibly and under-qualified advice.

Speaking With A Medical Professional

Speak with a medical expert, such as a qualified nutritionist or your primary care physician, before incorporating Coenzyme Q10 supplements into your daily routine. This is particularly crucial if you use medication, have underlying medical issues, or have particular health concerns. A medical professional can examine your present state of health, as well as your specific needs, to decide if taking CoQ10 supplements is right for you.

Your healthcare provider can explain any possible hazards or interactions with any medications you may be taking, as well as assist you in understanding the potential benefits of CoQ10. Additionally, they may assist you in figuring out which dosage and kind of CoQ10—ubiquinone or ubiquinol—is optimal for your unique set of circumstances and health objectives. The advice of a healthcare professional is quite helpful in making sure that CoQ10 enhances your current health regimen without having any unwanted side effects.

Establishing a Supplementary Program

After speaking with a medical expert and getting their advice, you may start formulating a Coenzyme Q10 supplement regimen specific to your requirements. It's critical to select premium CoQ10 products from reliable suppliers because supplement potency and purity can differ. Seek for goods that satisfy set criteria and have undergone independent quality testing.

Your healthcare provider's advice and your own health goals will determine the appropriate dosage and frequency of CoQ10 supplementation. While some people use CoQ10 regularly, others might only do so infrequently. Adhering to the recommended dosage is essential for obtaining the intended health advantages.

Including CoQ10 in your daily routine is not too difficult. It's convenient to take with a glass of water because it's frequently sold as soft gels or capsules. You can take CoQ10 with or without meals, though some people find that taking it with a meal improves absorption.

Tracking Your Development

Including Coenzyme Q10 in your daily routine requires regular monitoring of your health and progress. Note any changes in your level of energy, general health, and any particular health issues you're dealing with.

At your follow-up sessions, discuss this information with your healthcare physician to make sure CoQ10 is producing the expected results.

It's also critical to be aware of any possible negative reactions or side effects. Even while CoQ10 is usually seen to be safe when taken as prescribed, some people may have slight side effects, such as upset stomach. See your healthcare practitioner right away if you experience any unpleasant or unexpected responses.

It is important to make an informed and deliberate choice when adding Coenzyme Q10 to your daily regimen.

Speaking with a medical expert makes sure that your use of CoQ10 supports your overall health objectives and doesn't conflict with other prescriptions or therapies. You may optimize the possible advantages of CoQ10 while putting your general health first by developing a supplement regimen based on their advice and tracking your results.

Every single cell in the human body contains the naturally occurring substance coenzyme Q10 or CoQ10. It functions as a potent antioxidant and is essential for the cellular synthesis of energy. Because of the possible health benefits, CoQ10 supplements have become more and more popular in recent years. They are frequently used to enhance many elements of well-being. We'll talk about a few commonly asked questions concerning Coenzyme Q10 supplements in this discussion.

What Is Coq10, Or Coenzyme Q10?

The fat-soluble substance coenzyme Q10 is found in the mitochondria, which are our cells' energy-producing organelles. It plays an essential role in the electron transport chain, which is in charge of generating adenosine triphosphate (ATP), the main source of energy for cells. Furthermore, CoQ10 possesses antioxidant qualities that aid in shielding cells from oxidative harm brought on by free radicals.

Why Do People Use Supplements Containing Coq10?

People take CoQ10 supplements for a range of purposes. Since CoQ10 is involved in the synthesis of energy required for the heart to operate properly, many individuals use it to promote heart health. Additionally, it might help enhance cholesterol profiles and lower blood pressure. Some people also take CoQ10 to prevent the signs of aging, increase energy, and support general health. Its potential benefits in managing specific medical diseases, like migraines and Parkinson's disease, have also been investigated.

Yes, coenzyme Q10 can be found in trace amounts in a variety of meals. However, organ meats like liver, kidney, and heart usually have the highest concentrations of coenzyme Q10. It can also be found in nuts, soybean oil, whole grains, and seafood, especially mackerel, sardines, and salmon. Although some CoQ10 is present in certain food sources, some people may need to take supplements to reach higher levels to address particular health issues.

Is it okay to consume CoQ10?

When used in the prescribed dosage range, CoQ10 is generally regarded as safe for the majority of people. Rare and typically mild side effects include digestive problems like nausea and diarrhea. However, as CoQ10 may interact with some medications, it's crucial to speak with a healthcare professional before beginning any new supplement, particularly if you have underlying medical conditions or are on any medications.

What Is The Recommended Coq10 Dosage?

The optimal amount of CoQ10 to take varies based on personal needs and health goals. A common daily dose for maintaining general health is between 100 and 200 mg. Nonetheless, larger dosages might be necessary for people with particular medical conditions or those taking medication under a doctor's supervision.

It's critical to adhere to the suggested dosage listed on the label of the supplement and speak with a healthcare professional to figure out how much is best for your particular situation.

How long does using CoQ10 supplements take to show results?

The length of time it takes for a person to notice benefits from taking a CoQ10 supplement varies depending on their unique circumstances. While some people may experience increases in their energy levels somewhat immediately, others may need to wait from weeks to months to observe improvements in their heart health or other illnesses. When using supplements, it's crucial to be persistent and patient because the advantages could build up over time.

Do CoQ10 supplements and prescription drugs interact?

Although CoQ10 is usually safe, there is a chance that it will interfere with some drugs. For example, it could affect how drugs that thin the blood, like warfarin, work. It's crucial to speak with your doctor before beginning a CoQ10 supplement regimen if you use prescription drugs, especially ones that are linked to heart health. This will help to prevent any potential interactions.

The use of coenzyme Q10 as a dietary supplement is becoming more and more common. It is an essential substance with several possible health advantages. But like with any supplement, it's crucial to use CoQ10 sensibly and in cooperation with your doctor to make sure it supports your health objectives and doesn't adversely affect any drugs you may be taking. To support any supplements, it's also critical to keep a balanced diet that includes foods high in CoQ10.

Upon

Actual Stories:

Coenzyme Q10, often known as CoQ10, is a substance that exists naturally in human cells. It is an important component in the synthesis of energy and a potent antioxidant. Although scientific studies have yielded significant insights into the possible advantages of CoQ10 supplementation, firsthand accounts from people who have included this supplement in their daily routines can illuminate its real-world implications.

Individual Testimonies:

A lot of people have had good results from taking Coenzyme Q10 supplements. A significant number of these first-hand accounts center on the enhancement of energy levels and general vigor. People have reported feeling less worn out, more energized, and better suited to participate in physical activities after taking CoQ10 supplements daily. This is consistent with CoQ10's basic function in the electron transport chain, where it facilitates the production of adenosine triphosphate (ATP), the body's main source of energy.

CoQ10 has also received recognition for its possible advantages to the heart. After taking CoQ10 supplements, some people with heart diseases have reported having better heart function and fewer symptoms, like shortness of breath or chest pain. These testimonies are consistent with research indicating that CoQ10 may improve heart health by increasing heart muscle efficiency and fostering normal blood pressure levels.

CoQ10 has garnered praise for its antioxidant qualities in addition to its effects on energy and heart health. Consumers have reported fewer wrinkles and signs of aging on their skin, indicating improvements in skin health. This is explained by CoQ10's capacity to scavenge free radicals, which are linked to early aging and skin damage.

Achievements With Coenzyme Q10:
Those who have seen notable changes in long-term medical conditions provide some of the most inspiring Coenzyme Q10 success tales. For instance, taking CoQ10 supplements has been shown to lessen the frequency and intensity of migraine sufferers' headaches. This may be related to the compound's ability to stabilize mitochondrial

function, which may be involved in the pathophysiology of migraines.

Furthermore, CoQ10 has drawn interest for its potential to help those with neurological illnesses including Parkinson's and Alzheimer's. Some people have talked about how adding CoQ10 to their regular routines improved their motor abilities, memory retention, and cognitive performance. Even though additional research is needed in this area, these success stories show that CoQ10 has potential as an adjuvant therapy for these illnesses.

Conclusion

An extensive array of possible benefits is demonstrated by firsthand accounts and firsthand testimonies regarding Coenzyme Q10 supplements.

These anecdotes corroborate the scientific data indicating the critical function CoQ10 plays in antioxidant defense, cardiovascular health, and energy production. People's stories are powerful, but it's vital to remember that everyone has different experiences and that everyone reacts differently to CoQ10 supplementation.

Before incorporating CoQ10 into your regimen, like with any supplement, it's imperative to speak with a healthcare provider, particularly if you have any underlying medical concerns or are currently taking other drugs.

Because Coenzyme Q10 interacts with some drugs, consulting a specialist is necessary.

The success and real-life tales about Coenzyme Q10 provide insightful information about the possible advantages of this supplement. CoQ10 has demonstrated potential in enhancing energy levels, heart health, skin appearance, and even managing specific medical disorders, even though it may not be a miracle treatment. These tales serve as a helpful reminder that achieving optimal health frequently entails several strategies, such as a well-rounded diet, consistent exercise, and, in certain situations, the addition of thoroughly studied supplements like Coenzyme Q10.